WHAT IS
PREGNANCY?

in the same series

What Is Sex?
Kate E. Reynolds
Illustrated by Jonathon Powell
ISBN 978 1 78775 937 4
eISBN 978 1 78775 938 1

What Is Menopause?
Kate E. Reynolds
Illustrated by Jonathon Powell
ISBN 978 1 78775 941 1
eISBN 978 1 78775 942 8

by the same author in the *Sexuality and Safety with Tom and Ellie* series

What's Happening to Ellie?
Kate E. Reynolds
Illustrated by Jonathon Powell
ISBN 978 1 84905 526 0
eISBN 978 0 85700 937 1

Things Ellie Likes
Kate E. Reynolds
Illustrated by Jonathon Powell
ISBN 978 1 84905 525 3
eISBN 978 0 85700 936 4

What's Happening to Tom?
Kate E. Reynolds
Illustrated by Jonathon Powell
ISBN 978 1 84905 523 9
eISBN 978 0 85700 934 0

Things Tom Likes
Kate E. Reynolds
Illustrated by Jonathon Powell
ISBN 978 1 84905 522 2
eISBN 978 0 85700 933 3

What Is Pregnancy?

A Guide for People with Autism, Special Educational Needs and Disabilities

Kate E. Reynolds

Illustrated by Jonathon Powell

Jessica Kingsley Publishers

London and Philadelphia

First published in Great Britain in 2022 by Jessica Kingsley Publishers
An Hachette Company

1

A CIP catalogue record for this title is available from the British Library
and the Library of Congress

ISBN 978 1 78775 939 8
eISBN 978 1 78775 940 4

Printed and bound in China by Leo Paper Products

Jessica Kingsley Publishers' policy is to use papers that are natural, renewable
and recyclable products and made from wood grown in sustainable forests.
The logging and manufacturing processes are expected to conform to the
environmental regulations of the country of origin.

Jessica Kingsley Publishers
Carmelite House
50 Victoria Embankment
London EC4Y 0DZ

www.jkp.com

With endless thanks to my daughter, Francesca,
for inviting me to be at her side as she gave birth
to my granddaughter, Mina.

Kate

Thanks to my mum, Kelsy Powell, for her love,
support and all the help through the years.

Jonathon

DISCLAIMER

Illustrations and wording in this book are explicit and focus on aspects of pregnancy and relationships. The author and illustrator are not responsible for any offence that may be caused.

The content of this book should not be regarded as a substitute for the advice of a medical or mental health professional practitioner or recommended therapy, treatment or professional consultation. The author and illustrator are not responsible or liable for any diagnosis made or actions taken based on the content of this book. Always consult your family doctor or licensed mental health professional if you are concerned about your health or that of a child or young person with autism, developmental and intellectual disabilities.

Research shows that many people who have autism or special educational needs and disabilities (SEND) have poor experiences of prenatal and postnatal care and high levels of stress, anxiety and depression.

Most first-time parents need to learn about pregnancy, labour and caring for a baby. The difference is in providing accessible teaching – repeating information in different practical, visual or easy-to-read ways to support understanding and allow time for this process.

Some people have planned a baby. It is important to ensure partners, who also may have a level of autism or SEND, understand antenatal care, pregnancy and childcare, so they can support each other and prepare for their baby.

Sometimes people worry that they will be forced to have a termination (abortion), so they don't see a doctor or tell anyone that they are pregnant. They may be in the later stages of pregnancy or even in labour before they ask for medical help. However, people with disabilities have the legal right to create a family, to have reproductive autonomy and to marry or enter a civil partnership, with very few exceptions.

As part of the *Healthy Loving, Healthy Living* series, this book uses explicit wording and illustrations. The wording is gender-neutral, so we use "parents" instead of "mothers" and "people" instead of "women". The purpose is to support and give confidence to people with autism and SEND through accessible pregnancy information, which they can read alone or with support.

Having a baby is an exciting time. Like all new parents, you need to learn about pregnancy, giving birth, keeping healthy and how to care for your baby.

Pregnancy happens when a penis ejaculates into a vagina during sex without contraception (something that prevents pregnancy, such as a condom). Millions of sperm spurt out and swim up into the womb and into the fallopian tubes. A sperm is too small to see but you can see the liquid it is in.

A sperm joins together with a human egg which moves along the tube back into the womb. It attaches to the womb, keeps growing and is the start of pregnancy.

Sometimes people don't know what sex is or they don't use contraception properly or they are forced to have sex (rape), so the pregnancy isn't expected. If this happens to you, you may keep your baby or end the pregnancy. You can talk to your doctor about what you want to do.

If the sperm and egg join in the fallopian tube and get stuck there, the egg can't grow properly so it has to be removed by an operation or medicine. If you are pregnant and have any of these things, contact your doctor straight away:

- Sharp tummy pain, usually down one side and when you pee or poo.
- Bleeding from your vagina.
- Pain in your shoulders.
- Severe dizziness.

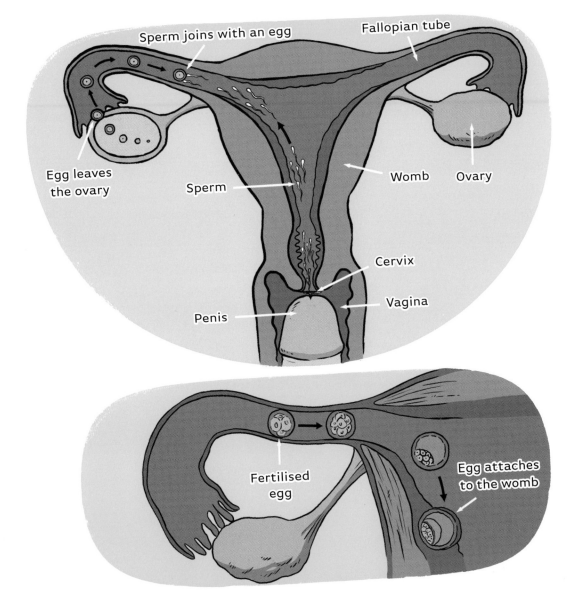

If you're pregnant, hormones in your body change and these things happen:

- Your periods stop. You might bleed a little bit when you're first pregnant, but then not again until after your baby is born.
- You may experience "morning sickness", which is feeling sick or being sick. It can happen any time of the day or night.
- You may feel really tired, like you've never felt before.
- Your breasts may hurt, get bigger and tingle. If you look in the mirror your nipples may stick out more and the dark circle on them (the areola) can look darker. You may see blue veins on your breasts.
- You may pee more, even at night. You might get constipated, which is when your tummy aches and your poo is hard and difficult to push out.
- More liquid than usual may come from your vagina. If it smells horrible, you should see a doctor.
- Lots of different things happen with your eating and drinking. You may hate food you usually like. You may be desperate to eat certain foods.

If you have sensory differences, you might feel things more than other pregnant people, like feeling sick (nausea). You can buy a pregnancy test in a pharmacy to do at home, but you must follow all instructions in the packet carefully. Your doctor also can do a test for you, if you think you're pregnant.

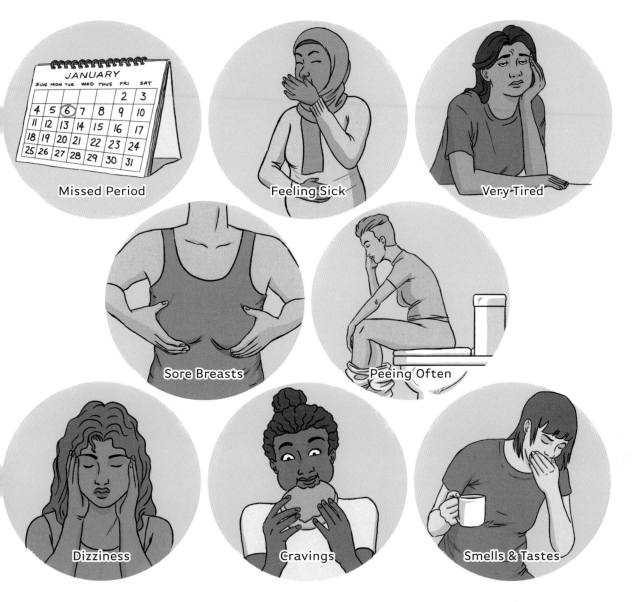

Missed Period

Feeling Sick

Very Tired

Sore Breasts

Peeing Often

Dizziness

Cravings

Smells & Tastes

If you are lesbian, gay, bisexual, transgender or questioning your sexuality (LGBTQ), you can still have children. If you or your partner have a womb, you can use a sperm donor, who gives sperm but not by having sex with you. The sperm is put into the womb by a doctor at a fertility clinic using a special medical tool.

If you are LGBTQ, you can have children by co-parenting too. This means you and your partner join with another person to get pregnant and parent children. This could be a gay couple of men with a single woman. The woman has a womb, so she can get pregnant using sperm from one of the men in the couple but not by having sex. The sperm is put into the womb at a fertility clinic.

There are lots of rules about getting pregnant these ways. A fertility clinic is there to help you and answer your questions.

A fertility clinic can also give you advice about who the children live with, how much each parent sees the children and who pays for childcare.

LGBTQ partners can also find a surrogate, which is when a woman gets pregnant with an egg and sperm from other people and allows the baby to grow in her womb. The baby is given to the LGBTQ couple after birth.

Some of these ways of having children are tricky. Your doctor can help you.

LGBTQ partners can also adopt and foster children.

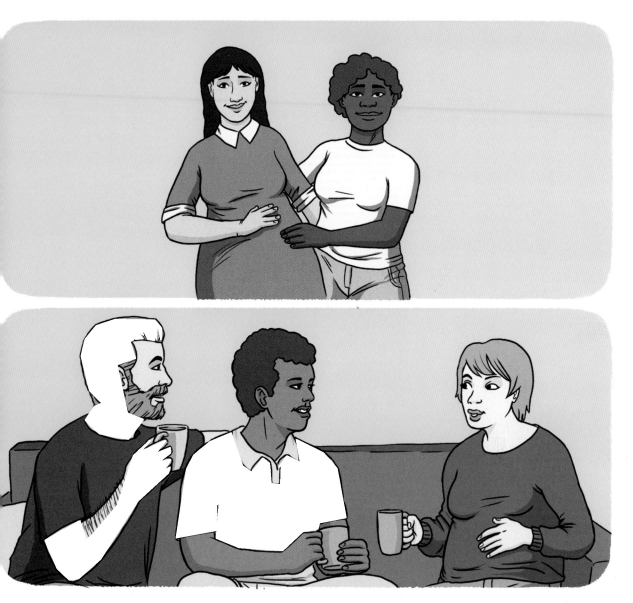

Midwives care for you when you're pregnant, when you're giving birth (called labour) and after birth. When you meet your midwife it's a chance to ask about things that are worrying you. You can explain your disability so you get support.

If you don't like crowded waiting rooms, you could ask to be the first appointment of your midwife's day. If your midwife is talking too quickly, you can ask them to slow down a bit. If you understand things better using pictures, signs or dolls, you can tell your midwife.

If you find change difficult, ask for clear advice about what's going to happen each visit. Sometimes things change quickly in pregnancy, especially in labour. If you find

stimming helps you keep calm, explain to your midwife how you stim, like rocking, leg shaking or finger flicking.

If you give birth at home (with a midwife there), you don't have extra sensory overload, like bright lights. If you give birth in hospital, your midwife can arrange for you to visit the maternity part of the hospital so you know what to expect.

You can take your partner with you. They can help you remember things and give you confidence. If your partner is also disabled, they can learn with you. The midwife will ask you lots of things about your health and support at home. If your relationship is abusive, your midwife can see you on your own and help you.

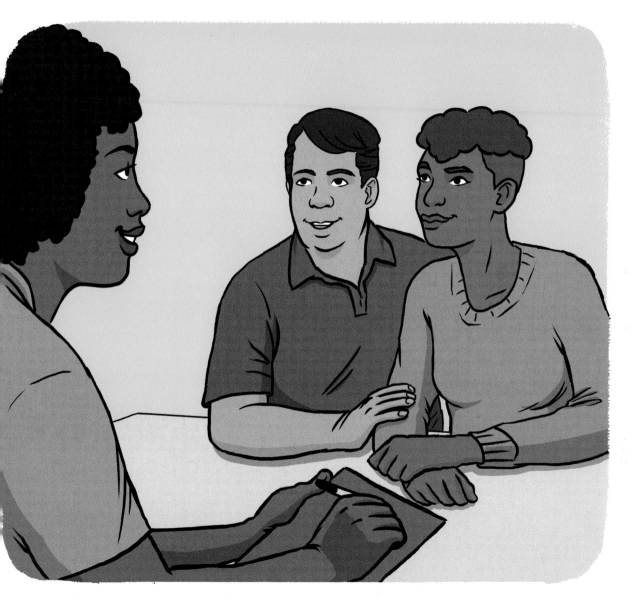

A pregnancy is counted in weeks and lasts about 40 weeks. Your midwife will work out the date when your baby is due to be born. Most babies are not born on their due date.

At around 12 weeks, you will have an ultrasound scan in a hospital. During the scan, jelly is put on your tummy and a scanner is moved over this. You can see black and white pictures of your baby on a screen. The scan doesn't hurt your baby or you.

By 13 weeks, your baby's organs (like the heart and liver), muscles, arms and legs and bones are all there. They just need to grow. Your baby floats in a sac of "waters" or amniotic sac in your womb. Oxygen and food goes from you to your baby in your womb from the placenta along a tube called the umbilical cord. This happens automatically.

From 16 to 24 weeks, you will start to feel your baby moving inside you. If you have sensory differences, the movement may make you feel a bit sick. As you get bigger you may get itchy, purple or brown lines called stretch marks on your tummy, thighs and breasts. They won't harm you or your baby and will fade after the birth.

At about 20 weeks, you have another ultrasound scan which shows the size and details of your baby's body. The scan shows if your baby seems okay. You may see another doctor or have a different test to check how your baby is.

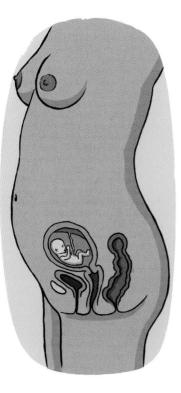

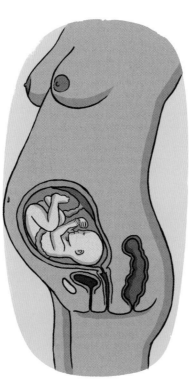

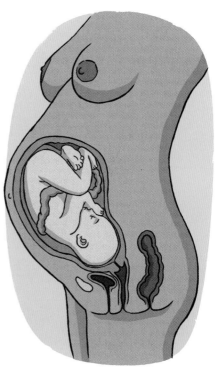

First Trimester
0–13 Weeks

Second Trimester
14–26 Weeks

Third Trimester
27–40 Weeks

There are lots of things you can do to help your baby grow and to keep yourself well. Your midwife can help you with this. Here are some suggestions for a healthy pregnancy:

- Stop smoking or cut back as much as you can.
- Stop using recreational (not prescribed by a doctor) drugs, like marijuana.
- Don't drink alcoholic drinks.
- Eat a balanced diet. Don't overeat as though you're eating for two people. Cut out foods that could harm your baby, like soft blue cheeses and meat that isn't cooked through. Your midwife can help you learn what foods to avoid.
- Cut down on drinks that contain caffeine, such as coffee and some fizzy drinks.
- Stay active.
- Wash your hands regularly. Wear gloves if you're cleaning up animal poo. Cook and store all food properly.
- Take folic acid, medication and vaccinations as advised by your doctor.
- Wear a good bra. Your breasts may get bigger and this can hurt your back and shoulders.
- If you feel worried, upset or can't sleep, or if you can't understand things about your pregnancy, ask for help.
- Your sense of smell, sight, sound, taste and touch may be stronger than usual, so you can ask your midwife for ways to feel better.

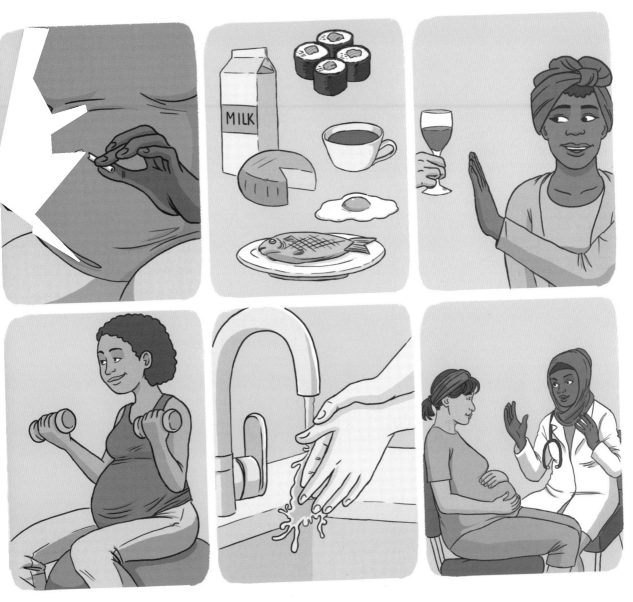

It's really important to have a midwife or doctor from early in your pregnancy, but it's never too late. This gives your baby and you the best chance of being healthy and well. This is the same for every pregnant person, but is especially important if you have medical conditions like epilepsy, diabetes or asthma. Your doctor will check your medicines. Don't just stop taking them.

It's a good idea to write down any questions you have for your midwife in case you forget. Your midwife will ask:

- To measure your baby bump with a tape measure.
- To take your blood pressure (by using a band that squeezes your arm).
- To test your urine. You will be asked to pee in a small pot in the toilet.
- To take blood from a vein in your arm to check you are well. If this worries you, speak with your midwife about it.
- To listen to your baby's heartbeat. Your midwife will use a stethoscope or a metal tool which feels cold.
- How you feel, what support you have at home, if you have a social worker or other support. This is also a chance to ask if there's anything you don't understand or you're worried about.

Your midwife may also refer you to the hospital for a scan of your tummy.

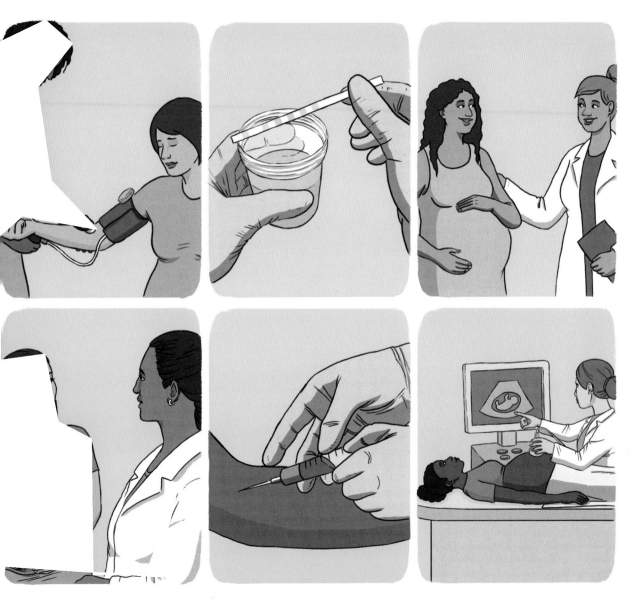

A birth plan is when you write down what you want to happen in labour to keep you calm and feeling okay. Think about:

- Who you want with you (including the midwife) to calm you when labour is tiring or there are sudden changes.
- Things that upset you, like loud noises, too many people in the room, bright lights or being too hot or cold. If you are going to hospital, you can bring your own things, like soft lights and music, to calm you.
- Massage, when someone rubs your shoulders or back to help you relax.
- A position that you want to give birth in, like kneeling, standing or lying on your side on the bed.

- Using a TENS machine. Small pads are put on your skin, which vibrate and make you feel tingly. This reduces pain but doesn't hurt your baby or you.
- A warm bath or shower which might help you feel calmer.
- What pain relief you want, like a birthing pool, painkilling pills, gas and air which you breathe in through a mouthpiece or mask, injected painkillers or an epidural, which is when a doctor puts painkilling medicine into your back. If you don't like needles or using a mask, talk with your midwife about this.
- If you want your partner to cut the umbilical cord. When your baby is born, the cord is cut and becomes your baby's belly button.

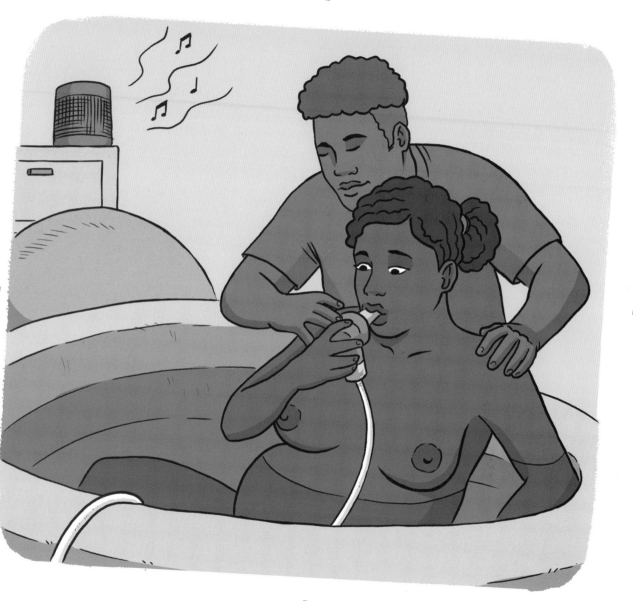

Midwives run antenatal classes before you give birth. You can ask them to repeat information or speak with them after a class to ask questions.

These classes give you a chance to meet other pregnant people and learn from each other, even if you just want to watch and listen. Sometimes you make friends with other parents and your babies can play together as they get older.

You can take your partner or a friend for support and confidence. They may help you remember what you've learned and they will learn with you.

Here are some of the things you learn in antenatal classes:

- What happens in labour and how your baby is born.
- Relaxation, including during labour.
- What to pack for you and your baby for delivery, if you're giving birth in hospital.
- Emotions and feelings in pregnancy and after birth.
- How to care for your baby, what your baby needs, how to hold your baby.
- Why your baby cries and how to work out what this means.
- How to play with your baby.
- How to feed your baby, breastfeeding, bottle feeding or a mixture. With sensory issues, you may find breastfeeding uncomfortable and messy, but parents with autism and disabilities can manage it with support.

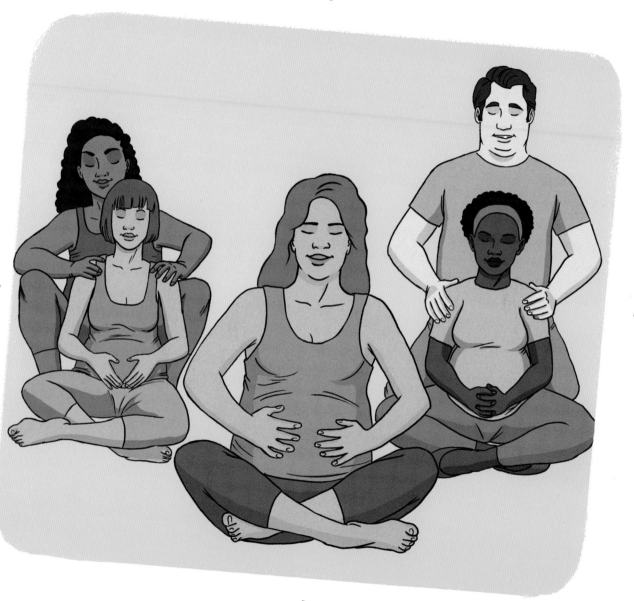

Sometimes there are emergencies in a pregnancy, so if you have any of these things, you should telephone your midwife straight away:

- Bleeding from your vagina.
- Itching feet and hands.
- Contractions – these are waves of pain over your baby bump.
- A change in your baby's movements.
- You have a high temperature of above 37 degrees Celsius.
- Swollen hands or feet.
- Severe headache.
- Your sight is blurred.
- Leaking liquid from your vagina.

Sadly, babies can die in the womb at any point in pregnancy. This is a terrible thing, but it doesn't happen often. Most of the time there is nothing that the pregnant person has done that causes their baby to die. Midwives can give support and find help from other people if this happens to you.

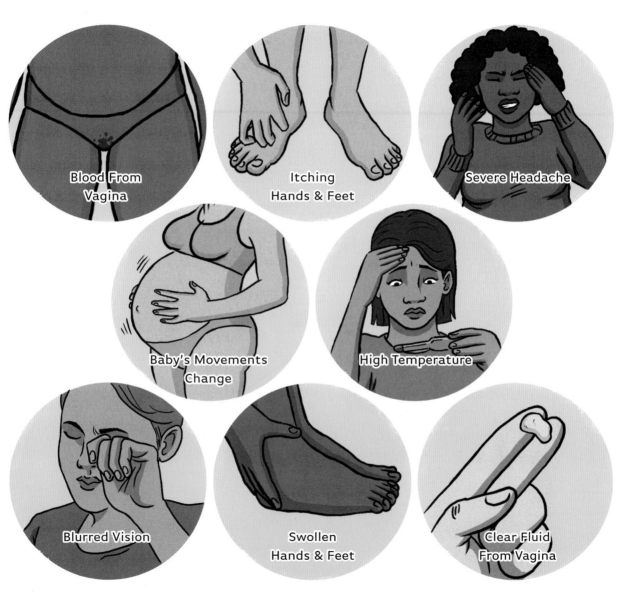

Like other pregnant people, when you go into labour these things may happen:

- Your waters break. This is when the sac of fluid, where your baby grows, breaks and the waters come out of your vagina. You should contact your midwife when this happens. You can't control the waters and it will be messy.
- You may feel discomfort or pain. If you have sensory differences, you may feel more pain or less pain than other people.
- You have an urge to have a poo, because your baby's head is pressing on your bowel.
- You have contractions, which are waves of pain across your baby bump. When you get about three contractions every ten minutes (you time them) or if they're so strong you need painkillers, contact your midwife.
- A "show", which is when some pinky, reddish, yellow or brown sticky stuff (mucus) comes out of your vagina.

If any of these things happen, you must telephone your midwife quickly:

- The mucus is green or smelly; this could mean an infection.
- Lots of blood at any time during your pregnancy.
- If you think you're in labour and you're under 37 weeks pregnant.
- Your baby is moving less than usual.

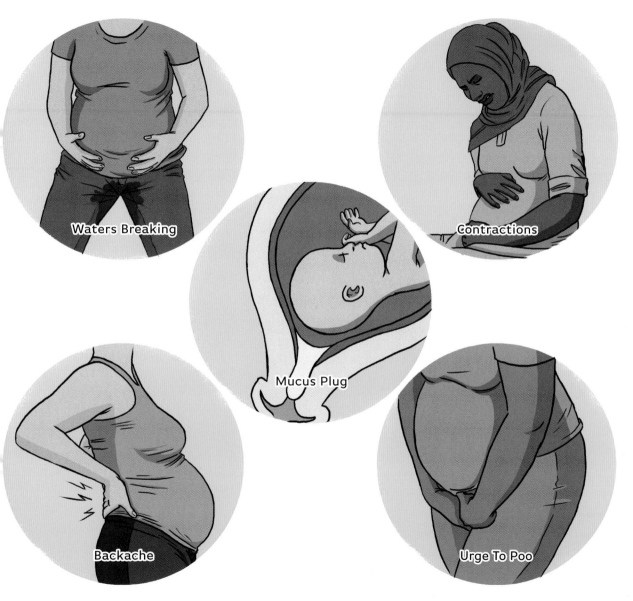

Waters Breaking

Contractions

Mucus Plug

Backache

Urge To Poo

Most of the time a baby is born through a vagina. This might seem impossible, but lots of things help this happen. For example, your baby has soft parts on the skull which allow the head to get smaller during birth.

During labour you might have a different midwife to the one you saw during pregnancy. They will support you and record your baby's heartbeat using a small hand monitor or two pads strapped to your bump or a small clip attached to your baby's head. These things won't hurt you or your baby.

Your cervix, at the top of your vagina, gets soft and opens out slowly until it is wide enough for your baby's head to fit through. Then your midwife will ask you to push downwards. Once your midwife can see your baby's head you'll be asked to stop pushing, so your baby can be born slowly and carefully. Labour can last hours.

If your skin is cut or breaks as your baby is born, this will be sewn up afterwards. You can have painkillers for this and something to numb your skin.

The umbilical cord has two clamps put on it, then it is cut in between the clamps. The clamps stop the cord from bleeding. After birth, your baby doesn't need the placenta, so it comes out of your vagina.

Giving birth is messy. There will be blood and fluid from the sac your baby was in and you might poo when you push your baby out. This is all okay.

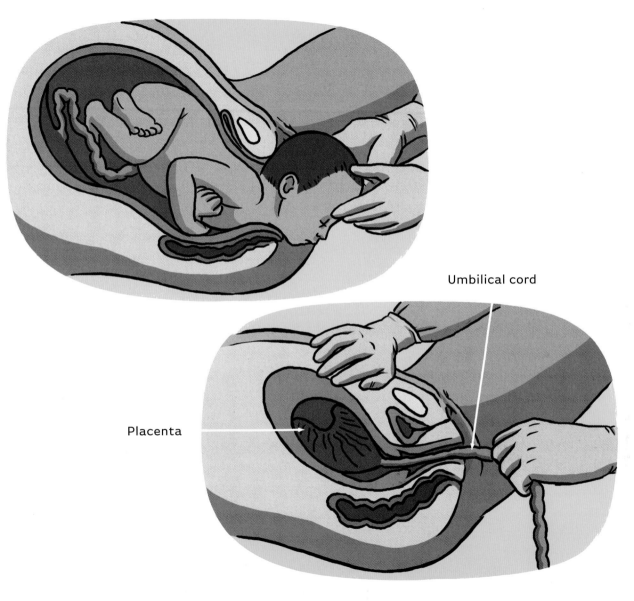

Umbilical cord

Placenta

Sometimes a baby is born by caesarean section. This is an operation when the doctor cuts across your tummy. It's a big operation but it may be done if:

- Your baby is breech, so your baby's feet or bottom are coming out first.
- Your placenta is very low, so there's a danger the placenta will come out before your baby or it will be damaged during labour.
- You have high blood pressure.
- You have certain infections, like genital herpes.
- Your labour is a bit slow or you're bleeding a lot from your vagina.
- Your baby isn't getting enough oxygen and food.

- Sometimes people have a planned caesarean section, which means you'll have a date when your baby will be born. You will be awake but numb from your waist down, so you won't feel pain. There will be a sheet across your middle so you can't see what's happening.

If it's an emergency, you will have a general anaesthetic (be put fully asleep).

It takes about six weeks to recover from a caesarean section. You will have painkillers, and you won't be allowed to drive or lift heavy weights until you see your doctor at the hospital after six weeks. You'll need help at home. The scar on your tummy will fade and usually is hidden under your pubic hair.

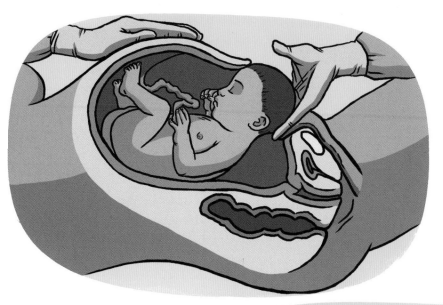

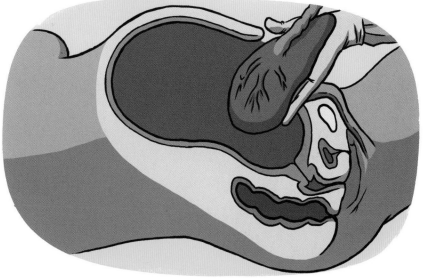

After the birth, the midwife will check your baby is breathing okay and will lay your baby on your chest. Most babies look a dark red or purple colour and have blood and vernix (the white stuff that protects your baby's skin in the womb) on their skin. Your baby's head may be a bit squashed due to the birth but this will change. This will be your first cuddle with your baby.

Once the cord is cut, the midwife will dry and warm your baby. The midwife will weigh your baby and put a band around their ankle with your name on it.

If you're in hospital you can have a bath before you go to the ward where you'll get support to feed and care for your baby. Babies cry for lots of reasons and you will get to know why your baby is crying.

When you go home a midwife and a health worker will support you to care for your baby. If you like your own routine at home, it might feel difficult because your baby won't have a routine straight away. You might feel exhausted, especially if you find it hard to sleep anyway. You can talk about this with your midwife or health worker.

There are groups where you can take your baby and meet other new parents. If you find this difficult because of crowds or anxiety, there are groups online. Talk with your midwife, health worker or support worker for help.

Remember that all new parents have a lot to learn and need support.

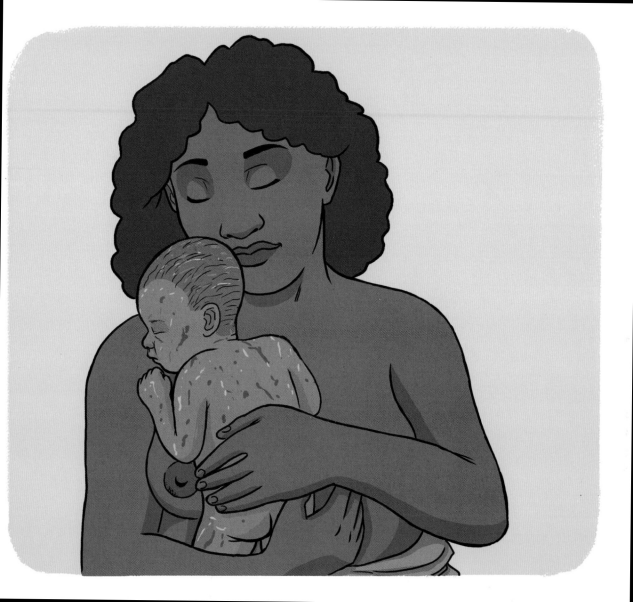

It's helpful to visit clinics and health centres before you have to use them.

Pharmacies can give you emergency contraception if your contraception hasn't worked or you didn't use any. You can buy a pregnancy test from pharmacy shelves without needing to speak to anyone.

You test your urine (pee) to find out if you're pregnant. There are instructions, but you may need a person you trust to help you use them.

A positive result means you are pregnant and a negative result means you are not pregnant. The instructions have pictures showing you what positive and negative results both look like.

Your family doctor can talk with you and refer you to other services. Your doctor may ask if you want to keep your pregnancy and what support you have. A pregnancy can be ended (called terminated or aborted), by taking medicine or by having a short operation in hospital.

It's important that you have this as early as possible in the pregnancy when it is safer for you. Your doctor can organize counselling for you to help you decide about your pregnancy. The choice is yours. No one can force you to end your pregnancy.

Sexual health clinics can refer you for a termination or abortion of pregnancy. You can also be tested for sexually transmitted infections (STIs).

Maternity services start after you have a positive pregnancy test. Pregnant people are tested for sexually transmitted infections (STIs) which could affect their baby. Sometimes you may need to take medication for an infection.

Name of service and key person	Address and phone number of the service	What does the service do?	How to find the service
For example: Highbrow Surgery Dr Agua	**For example:** 95 Douglass Lane Maisie GR1 4AN 09898 989890	**For example:** Pregnancy test and talk.	**For example:** Bus X58 to library. GP surgery is over the road with yellow handles on doors. Make appointment first.

HOW TO MAKE AN APPOINTMENT

- Write down dates when you're free to have an appointment in the next few weeks. Write down your phone number because the service may text you with your appointment.
- When you phone, tell the person speaking to you what difference you have, such as autism. This helps them support you and give you more time, if you need it.
- If you prefer a woman or man doctor, you can say so. You don't have to say why you want an appointment, but it can help the person to work out how quickly to get your appointment.
- Write the appointment down immediately and repeat it back to the person on the phone so you get it right.

WHAT TO SAY IN AN APPOINTMENT

It's a good idea to write notes about what you want to ask because lots of people get nervous and forget what to ask. Think about:

- Asking who needs to know about your appointment, any tests and results. There may be people you don't want to know.
- Have you had some sort of sex? What happened? Did you consent (agree) to the sex you had? Did you use contraception?
- How to explain why you think you're pregnant. For example, "I haven't had a period for six weeks", "I feel sick".

WHO CAN YOU TRUST TO TALK TO?

Remember that people might have to tell someone else what you say, if they think you might hurt yourself or someone else.

Name and how you know them	Phone number	Address	How to meet them
Family For example: My brother's wife, Molly	**For example:** 09876 543210	**For example:** 84 Long Leigh, Petalex	**For example:** Train to Petalex main station. Walk to Molly and Mark's house.
Friends			
Support worker			
Social worker			
Teacher			
Helplines			

Kate E. Reynolds, MDS, PGDC, PGDHE, BSC (Hons) SA, RGN, is a mother to two children on the autism spectrum, one of whom has intellectual disabilities. She worked for the UK's National Health Service for 18 years, much of which was in HIV and sexual health. Kate has written 12 books, most published by Jessica Kingsley Publishers and almost all about aspects of relationships and sexuality. She works closely with parents, caregivers and health educators, as a public speaker, trainer, advisor and researcher.

Kate can be accessed through her websites at **www.kateereynolds.com** or **www.autismagonyaunt.com**

Jonathon Powell lives in Brisbane, Australia and has a Diploma in Fine Art and Bachelor of Animation from Griffith University, Queensland. He has illustrated for the *Sexuality and Safety with Tom and Ellie* six-book series by Kate E. Reynolds, *Can I tell you about Pathological Demand Avoidance syndrome?* by Ruth Fidler and Phil Christie and *Making Sense of Sex* by Sarah Attwood, all published by Jessica Kingsley Publishers. He provided artwork and animations for Family Planning Queensland. Jonathon also illustrated *What are... Relationships?* by Kate E. Reynolds.